Scientific Publishing Ltd. ™

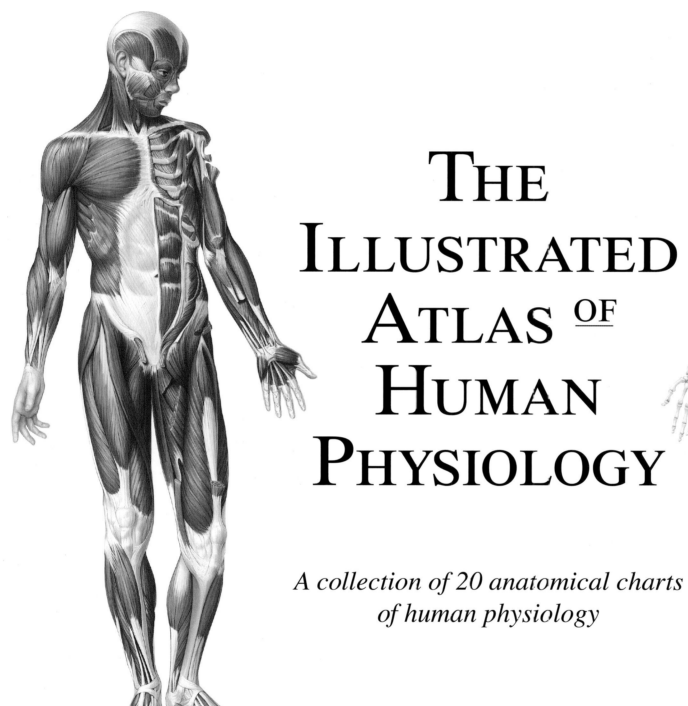

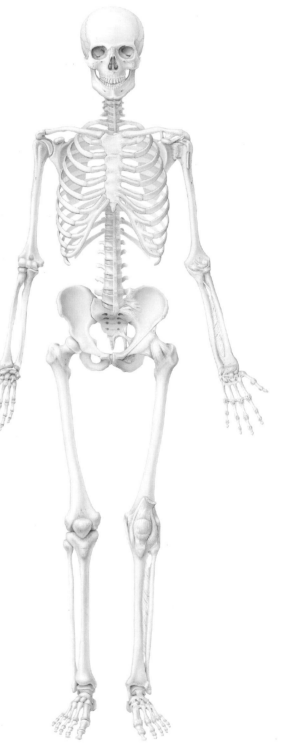

THE ILLUSTRATED ATLAS OF HUMAN PHYSIOLOGY

A collection of 20 anatomical charts of human physiology

Scientific Publishing Ltd.
www.scientificpublishing.com

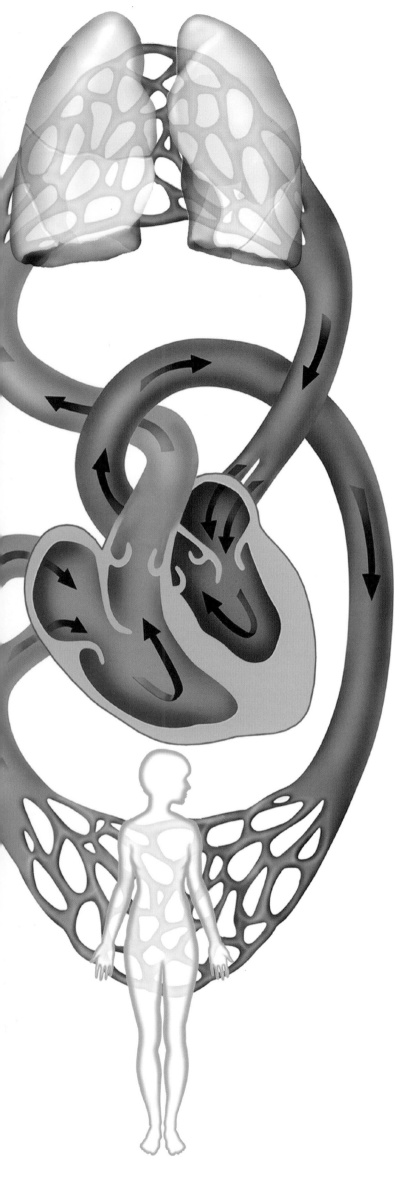

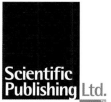

Scientific Publishing Ltd.

ISBN13: 978-1-932922-98-1   Item# PHYS-20

Published in the United States by: Scientific Publishing Ltd. 129 Joey Drive, Elk Grove Village, IL 60007

Printed in Korea

Individual chart titles are available at www.scientificpublishing.com

The Cardiac Cycle

Electrical pathways

The steady beating of the heart is regulated by electrical impulses traveling through the heart. The impulses originate in the sinoatrial node, also known as the body's pacemaker. The impulses spread across the atria, causing them to contract. Next the impulses travel to the atrioventricular node, pause, then spread through the ventricles along special conduction pathways called **bundle branches** and **Purkinje fibers**. This causes the ventricles to contract.

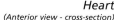

Sinoatrial node
Atrioventricular node
Atrioventricular bundle
Bundle branches
Purkinje fibers

Heart
(Anterior view - cross-section)

Electrocardiogram

An **electrocardiogram** (ECG or EKG) graphically records the electrical activity of the heart. A typical ECG records three waves, each representing different phases in the cardiac cycle.

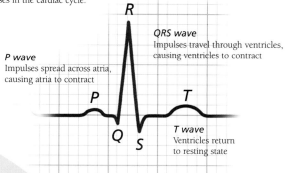

P wave
Impulses spread across atria, causing atria to contract

QRS wave
Impulses travel through ventricles, causing ventricles to contract

T wave
Ventricles return to resting state

R
P
Q S
T

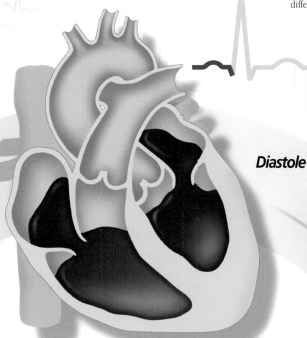

Diastole

Systole

Blood returns to the heart and flows into the atria. The pressure of the blood forces the AV valves open, and blood flows into the ventricles. The atria contract, forcing additional blood into the ventricles.

Diastole

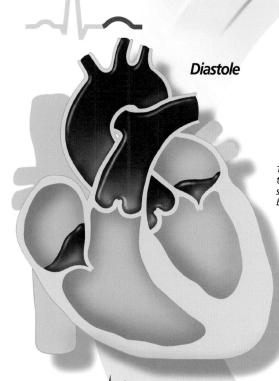

The ventricles relax, causing pressure in the ventricles to fall. Blood flowing back from the arteries closes the semilunar valves, causing the second heart sound. Blood begins to fill the atria again, and the cycle repeats.

The atria relax and the ventricles begin to contract. Pressure rises in the ventricles, closing the AV valves. This closure causes the first heart sound.

Pressure continues to rise in the ventricles until it exceeds pressure in the arteries. Blood is forced out through the semilunar valves into the aorta and pulmonary trunk.

Heart sound **dub**

Heart sound **lub**

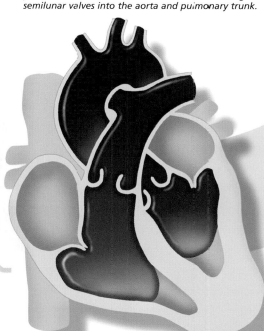

Systole

Heart
(Section view)

Superior vena cava
Pulmonary semilunar valve
Right atrium
Tricuspid (right AV) valve
Inferior vena cava
Aorta
Left pulmonary artery
Left atrium
Bicuspid (left AV) valve
Aortic semilunar valve
Left ventricle
Right ventricle

PLATE 1

The Digestive Process

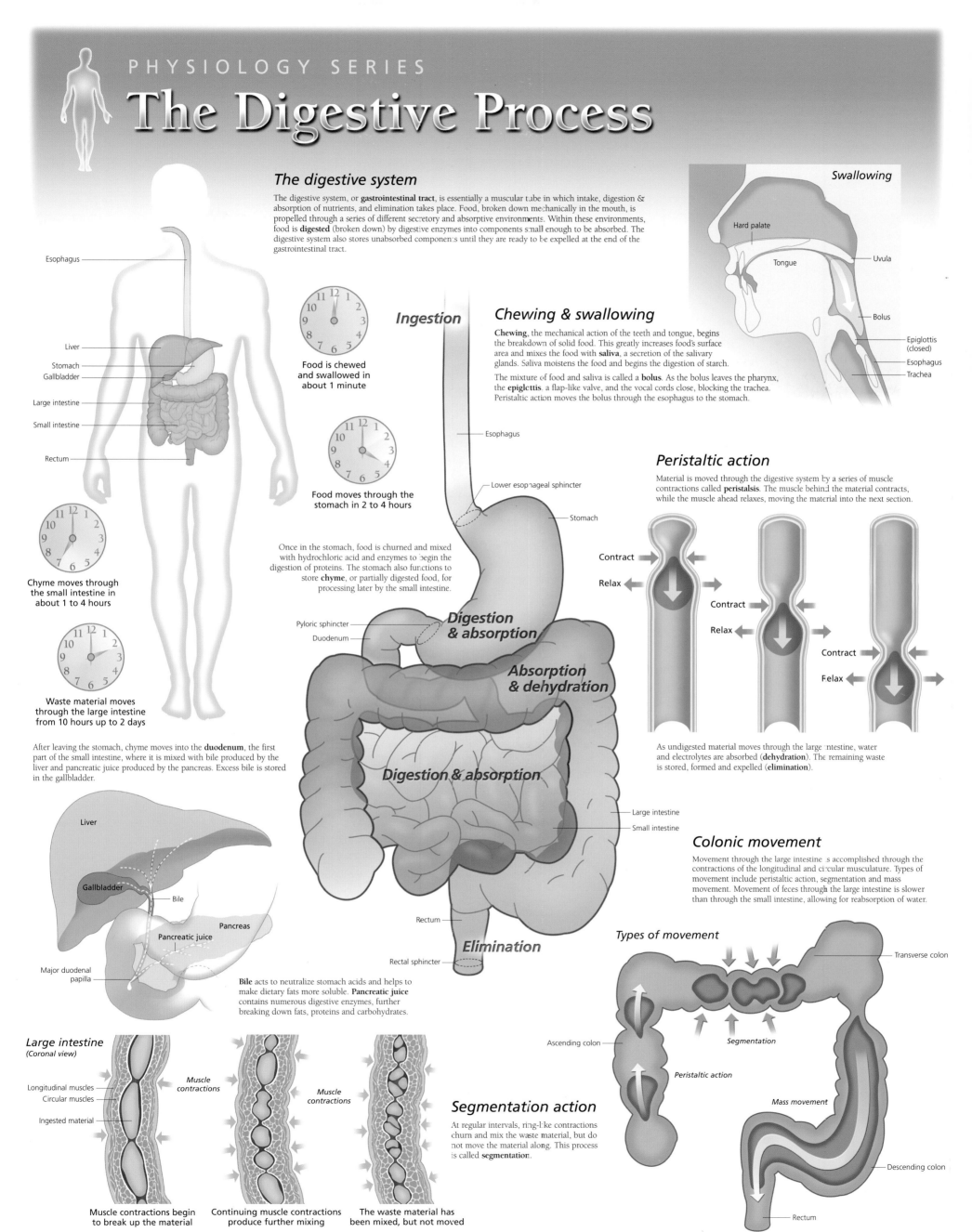

The digestive system

The digestive system, or **gastrointestinal tract**, is essentially a muscular tube in which intake, digestion & absorption of nutrients, and elimination takes place. Food, broken down mechanically in the mouth, is propelled through a series of different secretory and absorptive environments. Within these environments, food is **digested** (broken down) by digestive enzymes into components small enough to be absorbed. The digestive system also stores unabsorbed components until they are ready to be expelled at the end of the gastrointestinal tract.

Esophagus
Liver
Stomach
Gallbladder
Large intestine
Small intestine
Rectum

Food is chewed and swallowed in about 1 minute

Food moves through the stomach in 2 to 4 hours

Chyme moves through the small intestine in about 1 to 4 hours

Waste material moves through the large intestine from 10 hours up to 2 days

Swallowing

Hard palate
Tongue
Uvula
Bolus
Epiglottis (closed)
Esophagus
Trachea

Ingestion

Esophagus
Lower esophageal sphincter
Stomach

Chewing & swallowing

Chewing, the mechanical action of the teeth and tongue, begins the breakdown of solid food. This greatly increases food's surface area and mixes the food with **saliva**, a secretion of the salivary glands. Saliva moistens the food and begins the digestion of starch.

The mixture of food and saliva is called a **bolus**. As the bolus leaves the pharynx, the **epiglottis**, a flap-like valve, and the vocal cords close, blocking the trachea. Peristaltic action moves the bolus through the esophagus to the stomach.

Once in the stomach, food is churned and mixed with hydrochloric acid and enzymes to begin the digestion of proteins. The stomach also functions to store **chyme**, or partially digested food, for processing later by the small intestine.

Peristaltic action

Material is moved through the digestive system by a series of muscle contractions called **peristalsis**. The muscle behind the material contracts, while the muscle ahead relaxes, moving the material into the next section.

Contract
Relax
Contract
Relax
Contract
Felax

Digestion & absorption

Pyloric sphincter
Duodenum

Absorption & dehydration

As undigested material moves through the large intestine, water and electrolytes are absorbed (**dehydration**). The remaining waste is stored, formed and expelled (**elimination**).

Large intestine
Small intestine

Digestion & absorption

After leaving the stomach, chyme moves into the **duodenum**, the first part of the small intestine, where it is mixed with bile produced by the liver and pancreatic juice produced by the pancreas. Excess bile is stored in the gallbladder.

Liver
Gallbladder
Bile
Pancreas
Pancreatic juice
Major duodenal papilla

Bile acts to neutralize stomach acids and helps to make dietary fats more soluble. **Pancreatic juice** contains numerous digestive enzymes, further breaking down fats, proteins and carbohydrates.

Rectum

Elimination

Rectal sphincter

Colonic movement

Movement through the large intestine is accomplished through the contractions of the longitudinal and circular musculature. Types of movement include peristaltic action, segmentation and mass movement. Movement of feces through the large intestine is slower than through the small intestine, allowing for reabsorption of water.

Types of movement

Transverse colon
Ascending colon
Segmentation
Peristaltic action
Mass movement
Descending colon
Rectum

Segmentation action

At regular intervals, ring-like contractions churn and mix the waste material, but do not move the material along. This process is called **segmentation**.

Large intestine
(Coronal view)

Longitudinal muscles
Circular muscles
Ingested material
Muscle contractions
Muscle contractions

Muscle contractions begin to break up the material

Continuing muscle contractions produce further mixing

The waste material has been mixed, but not moved

PLATE 2

Skin Growth & Repair

Inside the skin

The skin is a highly elastic organ covering the entire outer surface of the body. It performs numerous functions essential to survival, including:

- prevention of fluid loss from body tissues
- protection against environmental toxins and microorganisms
- reception of heat, cold and pain sensations
- regulation of normal body temperature
- maintenance of calcium levels.

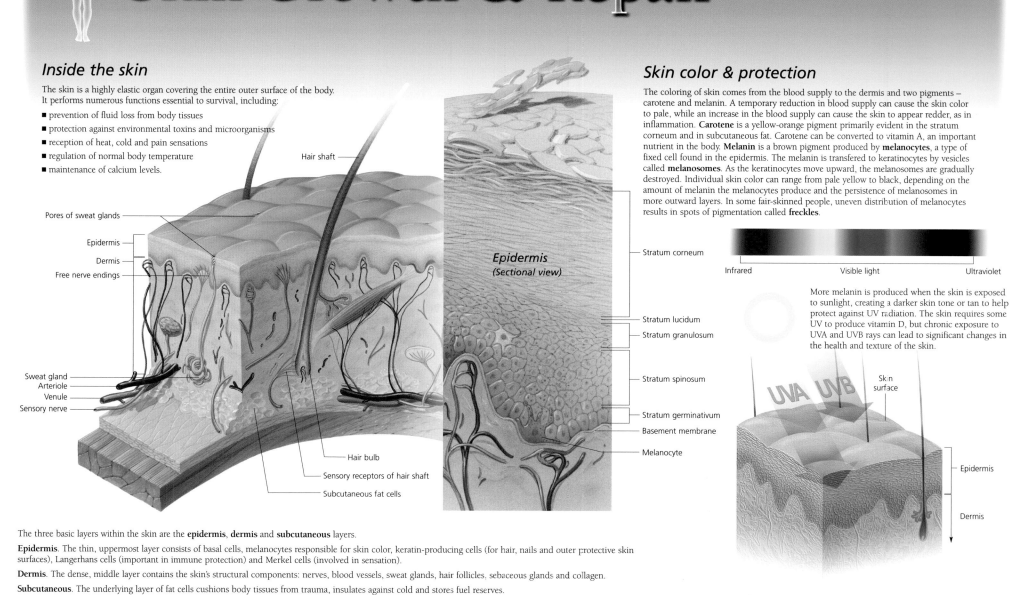

Hair shaft

Pores of sweat glands
Epidermis
Dermis
Free nerve endings

Sweat gland
Arteriole
Venule
Sensory nerve

Hair bulb
Sensory receptors of hair shaft
Subcutaneous fat cells

Epidermis
(Sectional view)

Stratum corneum
Stratum lucidum
Stratum granulosum
Stratum spinosum
Stratum germinativum
Basement membrane
Melanocyte

The three basic layers within the skin are the **epidermis**, **dermis** and **subcutaneous** layers.

Epidermis. The thin, uppermost layer consists of basal cells, melanocytes responsible for skin color, keratin-producing cells (for hair, nails and outer protective skin surfaces), Langerhans cells (important in immune protection) and Merkel cells (involved in sensation).

Dermis. The dense, middle layer contains the skin's structural components: nerves, blood vessels, sweat glands, hair follicles, sebaceous glands and collagen.

Subcutaneous. The underlying layer of fat cells cushions body tissues from trauma, insulates against cold and stores fuel reserves.

Skin color & protection

The coloring of skin comes from the blood supply to the dermis and two pigments – carotene and melanin. A temporary reduction in blood supply can cause the skin color to pale, while an increase in the blood supply can cause the skin to appear redder, as in inflammation. **Carotene** is a yellow-orange pigment primarily evident in the stratum corneum and in subcutaneous fat. Carotene can be converted to vitamin A, an important nutrient in the body. **Melanin** is a brown pigment produced by **melanocytes**, a type of fixed cell found in the epidermis. The melanin is transfered to keratinocytes by vesicles called **melanosomes**. As the keratinocytes move upward, the melanosomes are gradually destroyed. Individual skin color can range from pale yellow to black, depending on the amount of melanin the melanocytes produce and the persistence of melanosomes in more outward layers. In some fair-skinned people, uneven distribution of melanocytes results in spots of pigmentation called **freckles**.

Infrared   Visible light   Ultraviolet

More melanin is produced when the skin is exposed to sunlight, creating a darker skin tone or tan to help protect against UV radiation. The skin requires some UV to produce vitamin D, but chronic exposure to UVA and UVB rays can lead to significant changes in the health and texture of the skin.

UVA UVB
Skin surface
Epidermis
Dermis

Skin growth

The skin growth cycle can take up to six weeks and begins with a process called **keratinization**. Basal cells in the lowest layers of the epidermis are pushed to the surface and produce a protective protein known as **keratin**. These keratinized cells gradually die and are sloughed off the surface of the skin. They are continually replaced by new keratinized basal cells.

Outer layer of skin
Stratum corneum
Stratum granulosum
Stratum spinosum
Stratum germinativum
Basement membrane

Stem cells in the stratum germinativum divide, and one of the daughter cells is pushed upwards to the stratum spinosum.

The cells differentiate into keratinocytes, each containing filaments. As the cells progress outward, the number of filaments increases, helping to tie the cells together.

The keratinocytes produce large amounts of keratohylin, accumulating in granules, and keratin fibers. As the cells die, the fibers, granules and cell membranes form a protective layer.

The stratum corneum consists of 15 to 30 layers of dead cells, interlocked from the previous layer.

The dead cells, usually grouped in large masses, are shed or washed away.

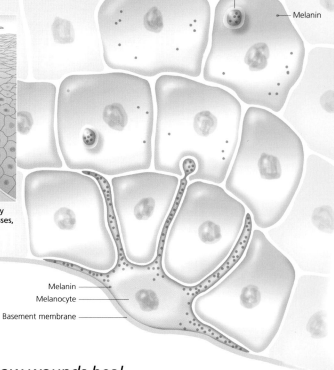

Melanosome
Melanin
Melanin
Melanocyte
Basement membrane

I. Wound

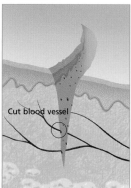

Cut blood vessel

II. Blood clot

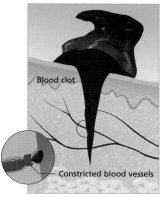

Blood clot

Constricted blood vessels

III. Scab

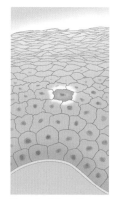

Scab

Exudate

Granulation tissue:
- Fibroblast
- Lymphocyte
- Macrophage

IV. Scar

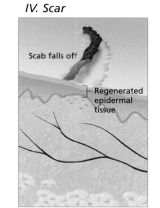

Scab falls off

Regenerated epidermal tissue

How wounds heal

After a wound occurs, the damaged portion of the skin begins to heal through a series of complex overlapping stages.

Initially a blood clot forms to stop bleeding and in most cases, dries to form a protective scab. Below the surface, inflammation takes place as nearby blood vessels enlarge and deliver oxygen and nutrient-rich blood and leukocytes to cleanse the site of dead tissue and bacteria. Rapid proliferation (regeneration) and migration of new epithelial cells help to replace the damaged area with new granulation tissue and close the wound. A scar is formed where the edges of the injured tissue grow together during healing.

PLATE 4

Bone & Bone Growth

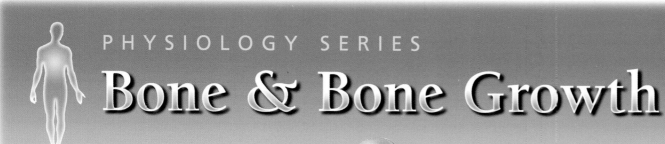

What is bone?

Bone is a living structure, constantly being built and rebuilt throughout our lifetimes. Our bones are strong, to support our weight, while being light enough to allow movement. Together with the teeth, bones store almost all of the calcium in our body. Red bone marrow, found in bones such as the sternum and femur, is a primary site of red blood cell formation.

Endochondral bone growth

Before birth, most of the skeleton is made of cartilage. **Osseus**, or bone tissue, gradually replaces the cartilaginous model. A narrow zone called the **metaphysis** separates the bone shaft, or **diaphysis**, from the end of the bone, or **epiphysis**. On the diaphysis (shaft) side of the metaphysis, cartilage is being replaced by bone. New cartilage is forming on the epiphyseal side. The combination of bone replacement and cartilage growth results in the bone growing longer.

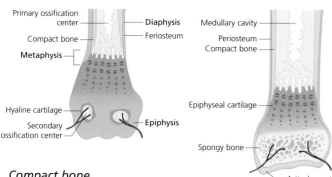

Primary ossification center
Compact bone
Diaphysis
Periosteum
Metaphysis
Hyaline cartilage
Secondary ossification center
Epiphysis

Medullary cavity
Periosteum
Compact bone
Epiphyseal cartilage
Spongy bone
Articular cartilage

Compact bone

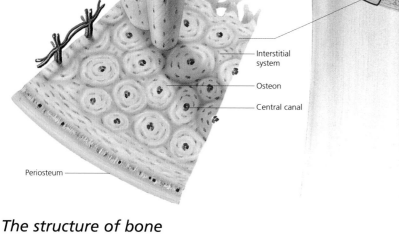

Lamellae (concentric layers)
Canaliculi
Lacuna (cavity)
Osteon
Osteocyte
Arteriole, venule and nerve in central canal
Lamellae
Spongy bone
Interstitial system
Osteon
Central canal
Periosteum

Femur
(Partial sectional view)

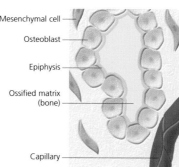

Periosteum
Medullary cavity
Periosteum
Compact bone
Nutrient artery in nutrient foramen
Yellow bone marrow
Diaphysis
Spongy bone
Epiphyseal plate
Epiphysis
Articular cartilage

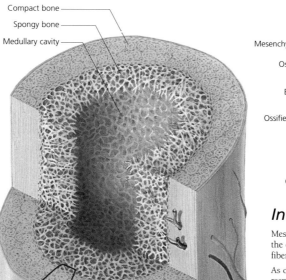

Compact bone
Spongy bone
Medullary cavity
Periosteum

The bone remodeling cycle

The process of bone remodeling continuously occurs throughout a person's life. Old bone is broken down and replaced by new bone.

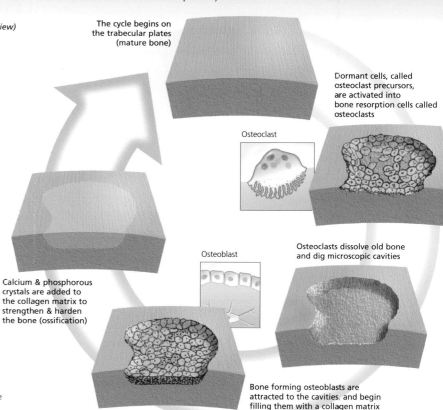

The cycle begins on the trabecular plates (mature bone)

Dormant cells, called osteoclast precursors, are activated into bone resorption cells called osteoclasts

Osteoclast

Osteoclasts dissolve old bone and dig microscopic cavities

Osteoblast

Bone forming osteoblasts are attracted to the cavities, and begin filling them with a collagen matrix

Calcium & phosphorous crystals are added to the collagen matrix to strengthen & harden the bone (ossification)

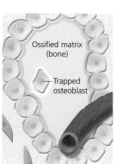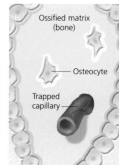

Mesenchymal cell
Osteoblast
Epiphysis
Ossified matrix (bone)
Capillary

Ossified matrix (bone)
Trapped osteoblast

Ossified matrix (bone)
Osteocyte
Trapped capillary

Intramembranous ossification

Mesenchymal cells differentiate into osteoblasts, which group together and begin secreting **osteoid**, the organic part of the matrix. Through the process of **ossification**, the mixture of osteoid and collagen fibers is hardened by deposits of a mineral composed of calcium and phosphates.

As ossification continues, some osteoblasts become trapped and differentiate into **osteocytes**, bone cells responsible for maintaining bone matrix. The bone grows outward, forming small struts, or **spicules**. The struts eventually interconnect, forming spongy bone.

Bone & calcium

Bone deposition and **resorption** (dissolution) occurs continuously through the process of bone remodeling. Even though calcium is constantly being removed and replaced, the calcium levels in the body are kept within a normal range. This is accomplished by hormonal action through negative feedback.

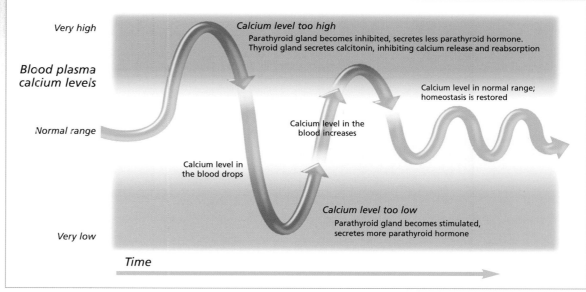

Very high

Calcium level too high
Parathyroid gland becomes inhibited, secretes less parathyroid hormone. Thyroid gland secretes calcitonin, inhibiting calcium release and reabsorption

Blood plasma calcium levels

Calcium level in the blood increases

Calcium level in normal range; homeostasis is restored

Normal range

Calcium level in the blood drops

Calcium level too low
Parathyroid gland becomes stimulated, secretes more parathyroid hormone

Very low

Time

The structure of bone

Bone is a type of connective tissue, with its own cells and an extracellular matrix. The **matrix** is composed of collagen fibers and mineral crystals made of calcium and phosphates. Bone cell types are:

Osteocytes — mature cells responsible for maintaining bone matrix

Osteoblasts — cells that secrete the organic parts of the matrix

Osteoclasts — multinucleate cells that dissolve bone matrix

Osteoprogenitor — divides to produce cells that differentiate into osteoblasts

The two kinds of bone are compact and spongy. **Compact bone** is relatively dense and forms the walls. **Spongy bone** is made of interconnected struts, combining strength and light weight. The center of a bone (the **medullary cavity**) contains bone marrow. **Red bone marrow** is a primary site of red blood cell formation.

PLATE 5

Muscle Action

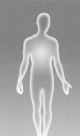

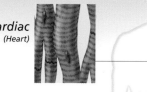
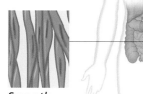
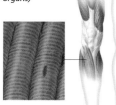

Cardiac
(Heart)

Smooth
(Digestive organs)

Skeletal
(Joints)

Muscles of the body

The muscular system interacts with the skeletal system to allow a wide variety of motions, including dancing, sitting and breathing. Muscles **contract**, or shorten, pulling structures together. Muscles can attach to bone (through a tendon), to skin or to other muscles.

Muscle action–smiling

One end of a facial muscle, the **zygomatic major**, attaches to the zygomatic bone. The other end connects indirectly to the corner of the mouth. When the muscle contracts, the corner of the mouth moves diagonally towards the cheek and we smile.

Another aspect of smiling is the contraction of the **obiculas oris** muscle, causing the skin under the eye to wrinkle.

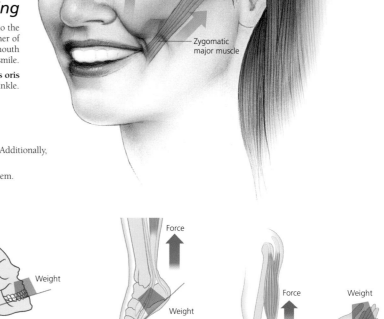

Obiculas oris muscle

Zygomatic major muscle

Muscle types

The three types of muscle are skeletal, cardiac and smooth.

Skeletal muscle provides the power that enables us to move under conscius control. Additionally, skeletal muscle provides the force needed to move venous blood back to the heart.

Cardiac muscle provides the overall force to move the blood through the vascular system.

Smooth muscle moves solids and fluids through the digestive system.

Skeletal muscle action

A skeletal muscle works by contracting, exerting a pulling force through a tendon connected to bone. In flexion the biceps brachii muscle contracts and the triceps brachii muscle relaxes, moving the lower arm upward. The muscle that produces the action is called the **agonist**, and the opposing muscle is called the **antagonist**.

This movement is reversed by the action of an opposing muscle. When the lower arm is extended, the triceps brachii muscle becomes the agonist, and the biceps brachii muscle acts as the antagonist.

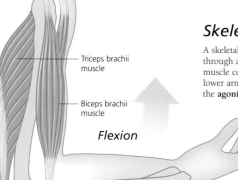

Triceps brachii muscle

Biceps brachii muscle

Flexion

Extension

Levers

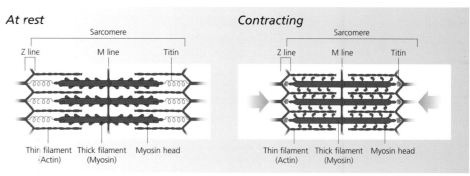

Force

Weight

Fulcrum

Class 1 lever

Weight

Fulcrum

Class 2 lever

Force

Weight

Fulcrum

Class 3 lever

Levers are structures that move at a fixed point, or fulcrum. Force is applied against a load or a weight. A lever, composed of muscle and bone at a joint, can change the direction, speed and distance of movement. Class 1 levers change the direction of the force, as in a seesaw. With Class 2 levers, a smaller force can move a larger load, but both speed and distance traveled are reduced. Direction remains the same. Class 3 levers move the weight in the same direction as the force. The gain is distance traveled and speed, but more force is required.

Skeletal muscle structure

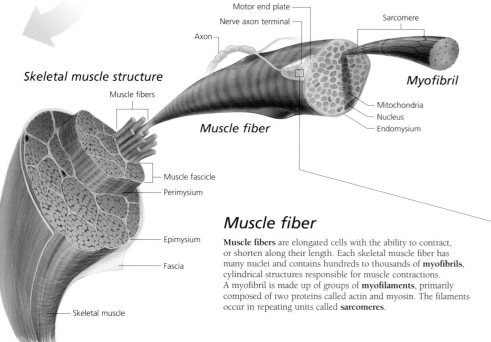

Motor end plate

Nerve axon terminal

Axon

Sarcomere

Myofibril

Mitochondria

Nucleus

Endomysium

Muscle fiber

Muscle fibers

Muscle fascicle

Perimysium

Epimysium

Fascia

Skeletal muscle

Tendon

Bone

Periosteum

Muscle fiber

Muscle fibers are elongated cells with the ability to contract, or shorten along their length. Each skeletal muscle fiber has many nuclei and contains hundreds to thousands of **myofibrils**, cylindrical structures responsible for muscle contractions. A myofibril is made up of groups of **myofilaments**, primarily composed of two proteins called actin and myosin. The filaments occur in repeating units called **sarcomeres**.

Skeletal muscle anatomy

Skeletal muscles are made up of muscle fiber bundles called **fascicles**, surrounded by the collagen and elastic fibers of the **perimysium**. Each fascicle is composed of muscle fiber cells, separated and supported by connective tissue fibers called the **endomysium**. The entire muscle is surrounded by a dense, irregular connective tissue layer called the epimysium. The epimysium, perimysium and endomysium come together to form a **tendon**, which attaches muscle to bone.

Sliding filament theory

At rest

Sarcomere

Z line   M line   Titin

Thin filament (Actin)   Thick filament (Myosin)   Myosin head

Contracting

Sarcomere

Z line   M line   Titin

Thin filament (Actin)   Thick filament (Myosin)   Myosin head

The sliding filament theory describes the mechanism of muscle contraction. In a myofilament the protein actin is found in thin filaments, and the myosin protein is in thick filaments. The myosin molecules have a free head and an attached tail. During a contraction the myosin heads attach to the actin filaments, then tilt, pulling the thin filament towards the sarcomere center. The myosin heads release, then attach to the next position on the actin filament.

Neuromuscular synapse

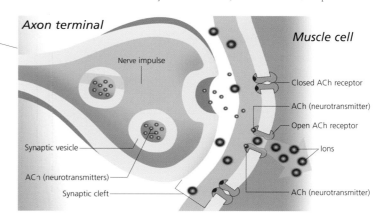

Axon terminal

Muscle cell

Nerve impulse

Closed ACh receptor

ACh (neurotransmitter)

Open ACh receptor

Ions

ACh (neurotransmitter)

Synaptic vesicle

ACh (neurotransmitters)

Synaptic cleft

Muscles contract when a signal from the nervous system travels through a **motor neuron** (a type of nerve cell) to a muscle cell. The nerve impulse moves through the neuron to an **axon terminal**, or synaptic knob. As the impulse arrives at the tip of the axon, synaptic vesicles merge with the terminal membrane, releasing "messenger" molecules called **neurotransmitters**. These molecules cross the tiny gap, or **synaptic cleft**, between the neuron and muscle cell. The neurotransmitter **acetylcholine** diffuses across the gap and binds to receptors on the muscle cell membrane, transferring the impulse to the muscle cell.

The effects of neurotransmitters are short-lived, because the cleft has to be cleared for future actions. The neurotransmitter molecules are either broken down by enzymatic action or reabsorbed and repackaged (**reuptake**).

PLATE 7

Vision

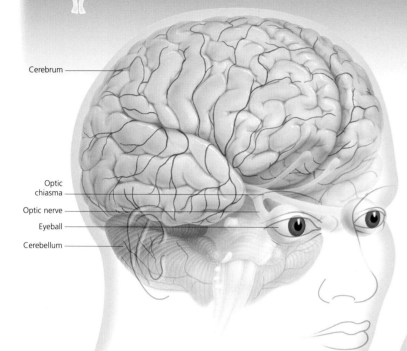

Cerebrum

Optic chiasma

Optic nerve

Eyeball

Cerebellum

Electromagnetic spectrum

Gamma rays	X rays	Ultraviolet		Infrared	Microwaves	Radio waves

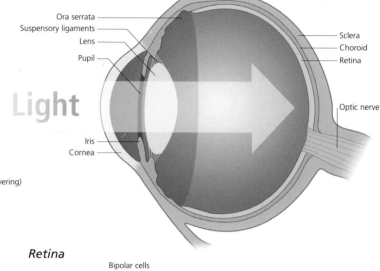

Visible light spectrum

The eye

The eye is one of the most important of our sensory organs. Often referred to as "the windows to the soul," the eyes are the organs which allow us **stereoscopic vision** (depth perception), an adaptation to the environment which ensured our survival. Our eyes receive a stimulus from light reflected off an object, and **photoreceptors** in the eye convert this light energy into nerve impulses. Only the visible light portion of the electromagnetic spectrum can trigger these photoreceptors. The brain interprets these signals and gives an accurate analysis of form, light intensity, color and movement.

Light

Eyeball
(Sagittal view)

Ora serrata

Suspensory ligaments

Lens

Pupil

Sclera

Choroid

Retina

Optic nerve

Iris

Cornea

Sclera (covering)

Pupil

Iris

Eyeball
(Anterior view)

Visual field

The **visual field** is the part of the external world that is projected onto the retina. The cornea and lens focus the right part of the visual field onto the left part of the retina of each eye, and the left part of the visual field is focused onto the right part of the retina of each eye. Within each eye the visual field is projected upside down and reversed because of refraction.

Retina

Ganglion neurons | Amacrine cell | Bipolar cells | Horizontal cell | Rod | Cone | Pigment layer

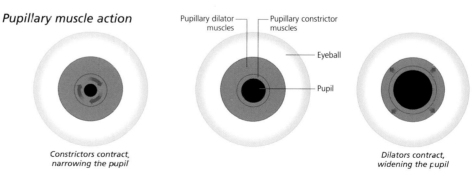

Light

Nerve impulse
(To optic nerve)

The retina

The **retina** lies principally in the back portion of the innermost **tunic**, or layer. There are two layers of the retina—the outer pigmented layer and an inner neural layer. The pigmented layer has several important functions, including the prevention of light scattering after it passes through the neural layer. Along with the **photoreceptors**, the pigmented layer assists in vitamin A cycling. The neural layer contains specialized neurons that act as photoreceptors—rods & cones. **Rods** respond to light levels rather than color, while **cones** respond to color and form. Bipolar neurons connect the rods and cones to the ganglion neurons. The axons of the ganglion neurons make up the optic nerve, which communicates to the brain.

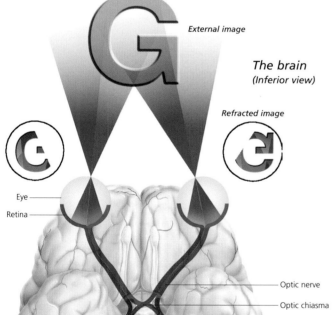

External image

The brain
(Inferior view)

Refracted image

Eye

Retina

Optic nerve

Optic chiasma

Optic tract

Projection fibers

Right cerebral hemisphere

Processed information received in the occipital lobe

Left cerebral hemisphere

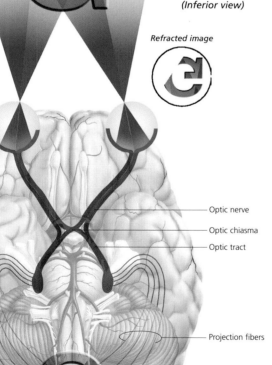

Pupillary muscle action

Pupillary dilator muscles

Pupillary constrictor muscles

Eyeball

Pupil

Constrictors contract, narrowing the pupil

Dilators contract, widening the pupil

Accommodation

The ability of the eye to keep an image focusing on the retina is called **accommodation**. When light enters the eye, light is **refracted** or focused onto the retina. In order to keep objects that are moving in focus, the eye has to adjust this refraction. It does this by changing the shape of the lens by use of the **ciliary body**. This muscular ring either contracts, making the lens less convex, or relaxes, making the lens more rounded or convex.

Visual pathways

Information about the visual field travels from the retinas to the brain. Information from the right side of the visual field travels from the left halves of both retinas to the left side of the brain. The signals from the left eye cross the **optic chiasma** to reach the right side of the brain. Information about the right side of the visual field hits the right halves of both retinas and travels to the left side of the brain — the signals from the right eye also cross at the optic chiasma. Within the brain, signals travel to areas responsible for perception and eye and body movements.

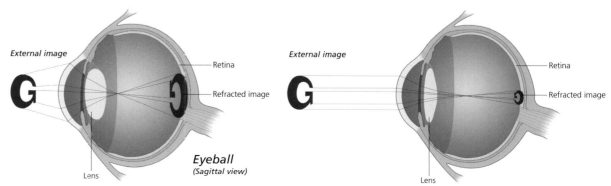

External image

Retina

Refracted image

External image

Retina

Refracted image

Lens

Eyeball
(Sagittal view)

Lens

PLATE 8

Hearing & Balance

The anatomy of the ear

The ear is a highly sensitive, complex organ containing the mechanisms for hearing and balance. The outer, middle and inner ear work together to collect, amplify and transmit sound signals to the hearing center in the brain. The inner ear contains the components responsible for detecting sound waves as well as the organs that detect the position and motion of the body, providing a sense of balance or **equilibrium**.

Helix
Antihelix
Tragus
Antitragus

Because they are located on each side of the head, the ears allow sounds to be localized from front to back. Recognition and analysis of sounds originating from side to side are processed by other mechanisms within the brainstem.

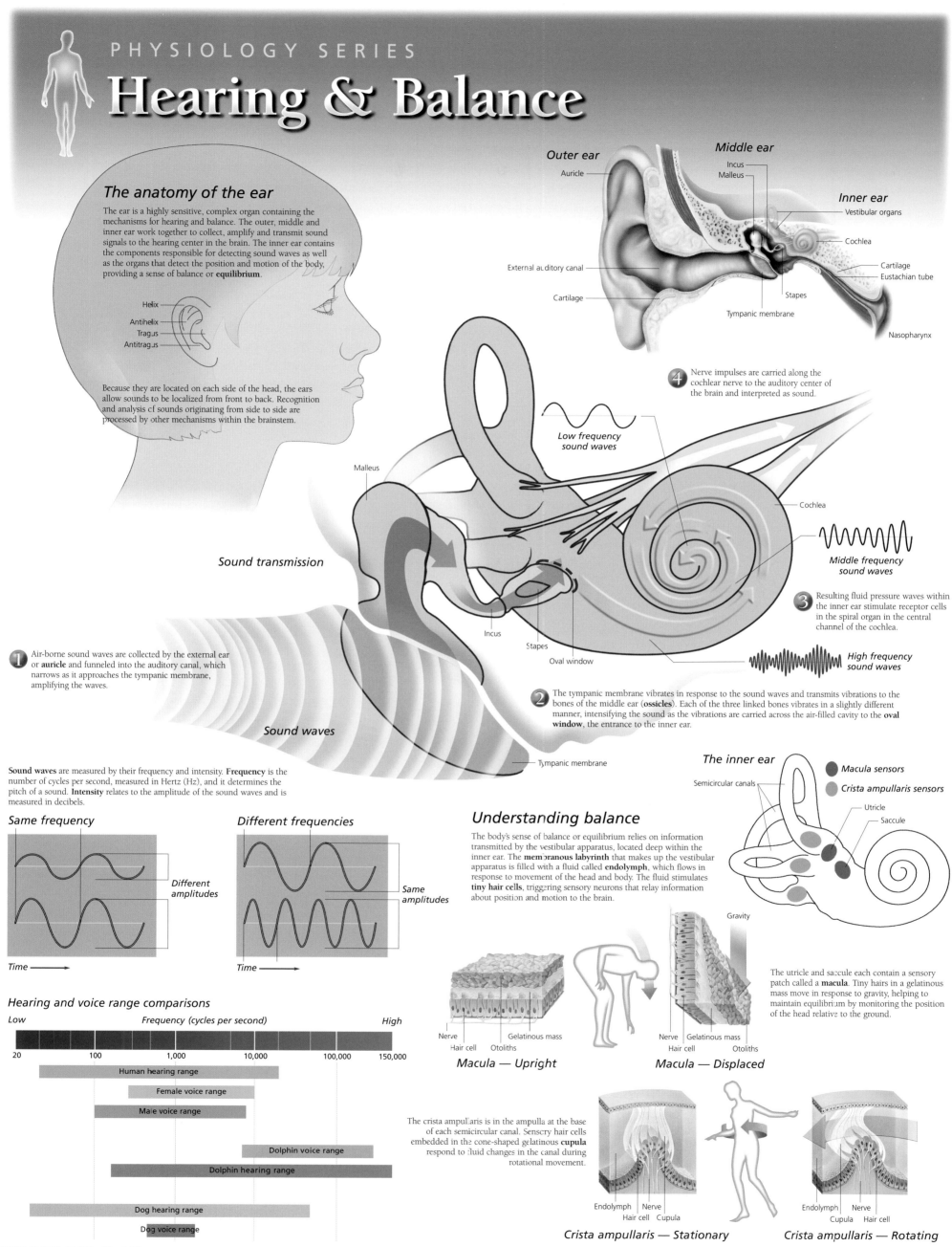

Outer ear
Auricle
External auditory canal
Cartilage

Middle ear
Incus
Malleus
Tympanic membrane
Stapes

Inner ear
Vestibular organs
Cochlea
Cartilage
Eustachian tube
Nasopharynx

Sound transmission

Malleus
Incus
Stapes
Oval window
Tympanic membrane

① ** Air-borne sound waves are collected by the external ear or **auricle and funneled into the auditory canal, which narrows as it approaches the tympanic membrane, amplifying the waves.

Sound waves

Low frequency sound waves

Middle frequency sound waves

High frequency sound waves

Cochlea

**④ ** Nerve impulses are carried along the cochlear nerve to the auditory center of the brain and interpreted as sound.

**③ ** Resulting fluid pressure waves within the inner ear stimulate receptor cells in the spiral organ in the central channel of the cochlea.

② ** The tympanic membrane vibrates in response to the sound waves and transmits vibrations to the bones of the middle ear (ossicles**). Each of the three linked bones vibrates in a slightly different manner, intensifying the sound as the vibrations are carried across the air-filled cavity to the **oval window**, the entrance to the inner ear.

Sound waves are measured by their frequency and intensity. **Frequency** is the number of cycles per second, measured in Hertz (Hz), and it determines the pitch of a sound. **Intensity** relates to the amplitude of the sound waves and is measured in decibels.

Same frequency

Different amplitudes

Time →

Different frequencies

Same amplitudes

Time →

Hearing and voice range comparisons

Low	Frequency (cycles per second)	High

20 100 1,000 10,000 100,000 150,000

Human hearing range
Female voice range
Male voice range
Dolphin voice range
Dolphin hearing range
Dog hearing range
Dog voice range

Understanding balance

The body's sense of balance or equilibrium relies on information transmitted by the vestibular apparatus, located deep within the inner ear. The **membranous labyrinth** that makes up the vestibular apparatus is filled with a fluid called **endolymph**, which flows in response to movement of the head and body. The fluid stimulates **tiny hair cells**, triggering sensory neurons that relay information about position and motion to the brain.

The inner ear

● Macula sensors
● Crista ampullaris sensors

Semicircular canals
Utricle
Saccule

Gravity

The utricle and saccule each contain a sensory patch called a **macula**. Tiny hairs in a gelatinous mass move in response to gravity, helping to maintain equilibrium by monitoring the position of the head relative to the ground.

Nerve
Hair cell
Gelatinous mass
Otoliths

Macula — Upright

Nerve
Hair cell
Gelatinous mass
Otoliths

Macula — Displaced

The crista ampullaris is in the ampulla at the base of each semicircular canal. Sensory hair cells embedded in the cone-shaped gelatinous **cupula** respond to fluid changes in the canal during rotational movement.

Endolymph
Nerve
Hair cell
Cupula

Crista ampullaris — Stationary

Endolymph
Nerve
Cupula
Hair cell

Crista ampullaris — Rotating

PLATE 9

Taste & Smell

Taste & smell

Two of our special senses are chemoreceptive systems: **gustation** (taste) and **olfaction** (smell). We depend on these senses for our survival, to know what's safe to eat and drink, to help identify friend or foe, to help us determine if our environment is safe or threatening. Both taste and smell involve **chemoreceptors**, specialized nerve cells that respond to molecules dissolved in fluid (mucus and saliva). The sense of taste is less discriminating than the sense of smell, and there is an overlap between taste receptors. The sense of smell is highly discriminatory, with several types of olfactory receptors, each responding to particular odorants. Taste interpretation is related to smell, texture and temperature, together with the taste bud sensations, but taste is profoundly affected by the sense of smell.

Upper respiratory tract
(Sagittal view)

- Frontal sinus
- Olfactory bulb
- Olfactory nerve fibers (CN I)
- Sphenoidal sinus
- Nasal cavity
- Tongue
- Pharynx
- Oral cavity

Olfaction

The sense of smell is called **olfaction**, or the detection of odors. Olfaction depends on specialized chemical receptors, or **chemoreceptors**, located within the olfactory epithelium. These receptors can respond to very small amounts of an **odorant**, a molecule than can be smelled. The brain integrates the input from several different receptors to identify a particular odor. Humans can detect about 10,000 odors.

As we breathe through the nose, the airflow across the nasal conchae produce turbulence, bringing airborne molecules into contact with the olfactory mucus. Sniffing increases the ability to detect odors by increasing the volume of air inhaled, which can intensify the stimulation of receptors.

Olfactory receptors

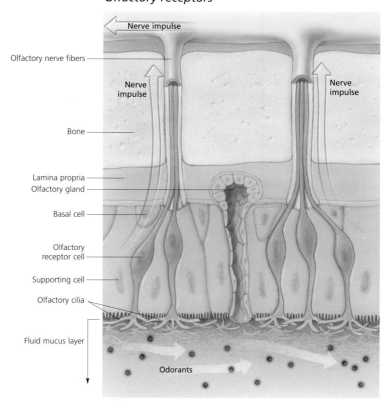

- Nerve impulse
- Olfactory nerve fibers
- Nerve impulse
- Nerve impulse
- Bone
- Lamina propria
- Olfactory gland
- Basal cell
- Olfactory receptor cell
- Supporting cell
- Olfactory cilia
- Fluid mucus layer
- Odorants

Concentrations

Taste sensations vary, depending on the **concentration** (the amount of a substance in a given volume or area). In low concentrations, bitter, sour and salty sensations may taste pleasant.

Graph:
- Y-axis: Sensation (Pleasant / Unpleasant)
- X-axis: Concentration (Low / High)
- Curves labeled: Sweet, Sour, Salty, Bitter

Lower concentration

Higher concentration

Olfactory receptors

Odorants dissolve in the fluid mucus layer, produced by the olfactory glands, then bind to receptor molecules on the olfactory cilia. The receptor potential that is produced travels along the axon to the olfactory bulb, which sends the signal to the higher brain centers. Unlike other senses, the olfactory neurons are connected directly to the cerebral cortex, rather than through the thalamus to the cerebrum.

Gustation

Gustation, the sense of taste, gives us information about the food and drink that we consume. **Taste buds** are the primary gustatory receptor, with each taste bud containing chemoreceptors called **gustatory cells**. Four basic tastes have been recognized: sweet, sour, bitter and salty. A fifth taste, glutamate or umami, has been reported. This flavor is associated with savoriness, as in aged cheeses or meat broth.

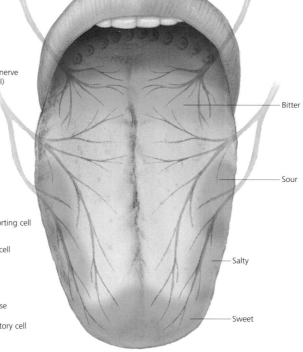

- Glossopharyngeal nerve (CN IX)
- Facial nerve (CN VII)
- Bitter
- Sour
- Salty
- Sweet

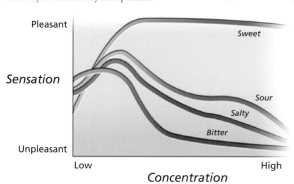

- Tastants
- Microvilli
- Supporting cell
- Basal cell
- Nerve
- Synapse
- Gustatory cell

The taste bud

Tastants, substances that produce taste, bind with receptor molecules on the surface of the microvilli. The resulting receptor potential travels to the basal end of the gustatory cell, where the impulse is chemically transferred across the synaptic cleft to another neuron. Gustatory cells last about 10 days, after which they are replaced by new cells generated from basal cells at the base of the taste buds.

Compared to sweet and salty tastes, we are 100 times more sensitive to bitter compounds, and about 1,000 times more sensitive to acids (sour). This may have a survival basis, since acids can burn the mouth and many toxins taste bitter. Typically an adult has more than 10,000 taste buds, but the number declines as we age.

The synapse

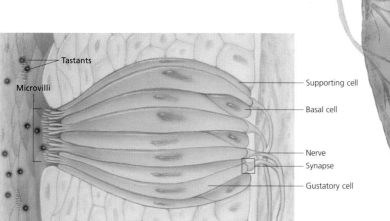

- Synaptic cleft
- Presynaptic cell
- Postsynaptic cell
- Impulse
- Closed receptor
- Open receptor
- Synaptic vesicle
- Neurotransmitter
- Ion

Neurons communicate with other cells at a **synapse**, the site of a nerve impulse transmission. The space between the **presynaptic**, or sending, neuron and the **postsynaptic**, or receiving, cell is called the **synaptic cleft**. As impulses arrive at the tip of the axon, the terminal bulbs release "messenger" molecules called **neurotransmitters**. These highly specialized chemicals carry nerve impulses across the synaptic cleft between the axon and the adjacent neurons or cells, either inhibiting or activating neural impulses in the target cell.

PLATE 10

Neurons & Neurotransmitters

The nervous system

CNS
(Central Nervous System)

Brain
Cranial nerves
Spinal cord

Spinal nerves

Ganglia

PNS
(Peripheral Nervous System)

Peripheral nerves

The brain
(Sagittal section)

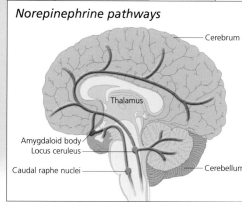

Cerebrum

Thalamus

Rostral raphe nuclei
Caudal raphe nuclei

Cerebellum

Serotonin pathways

Norepinephrine pathways

Cerebrum

Thalamus

Amygdaloid body
Locus ceruleus

Caudal raphe nuclei

Cerebellum

The nervous system

The nervous system is composed of two integrated subdivisions that are responsible for conducting and processing sensory and motor information: the central nervous system (CNS) and the peripheral nervous system (PNS), which connects the CNS to the rest of the body.

The **CNS** includes the brain and spinal cord, which are covered by protective membranes called **meninges** (dura mater, arachnoid and pia mater). The brain processes and coordinates all neural signals received from the spinal cord as well as its own nerves, such as the olfactory and optic nerves. It also performs complex mental functions such as thinking and learning.

The **PNS** transmits input gathered from the sensory organs to the CNS. Motor output signals are relayed back to the PNS and on to the body's muscles and glands. The PNS has three separate divisions called the autonomic, sensory and motor nervous systems.

The functional units of the nervous system are neurons.

Sensory neurons communicate information from sensory receptors to the CNS.

Motor neurons relay signals from the CNS to effector (muscle and gland) cells.

Interneurons coordinate and integrate sensory inputs and motor outputs.

Glial cells also make up a significant portion of the nervous system and provide important support for neuron activity.

The central nervous system (CNS) contains thousands of input and output connections between neurons that form dense networks within the brain. Synaptic connections are the tiny spaces between individual neurons where messenger chemicals called **neurotransmitters** are exchanged, initiating new electrical currents within target cells.

Neurotransmitters

Neurotransmitters are highly specialized chemical messengers that carry impulses across tiny spaces between **neurons** (nerve cells) in the body. The impulses are sent by the axon of one presynaptic nerve cell and received by the dendrite of the postsynaptic cell. Neurotransmitters are secreted at the contact points between these cells (**synapses**) and trigger receptors on the dendrite to inhibit or excite neural impulses in the target cell. Each type of neurotransmitter (such as dopamine and serotonin) has unique characteristics that allow it to bind to specific receptor sites on target cells.

Motor neurons transmit impulses to other cells, specifically muscle fibers or glands. Each neuron consists of a central cell body with a nucleus and numerous fiber-like extensions called **dendrites** that collect and relay information to the cell body for processing.

Dendrites

Nucleus
Cell body

Motor neuron

Integration

Myelin sheath
Axon

Impulse conduction

Nerve signals directed from the cell body travel towards target cells via the **axon**, a long extension of the cell membrane. An insulating **myelin sheath** made up of lipid-like Schwann cells insulates the axon. Spaces between these cells are called **myelin sheath gaps** (nodes of Ranvier). The axon branches into terminal fibers, which end in presynaptic knobs where neurotransmitter molecules are stored.

Myelin sheath gap
(Node of Ranvier)

The chemical synapse

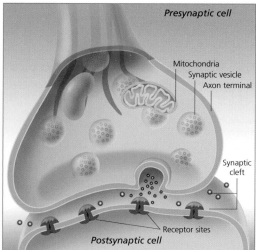

Presynaptic cell

Mitochondria
Synaptic vesicle
Axon terminal

Synaptic cleft

Receptor sites
Postsynaptic cell

Release of neurotransmitters

Neurotransmitter molecules are synthesized in the cell body or axon terminal, then packaged in sacs called vesicles. In a process called exocytosis, the synaptic vesicle membrane fuses with the axon membrane, and the neurotransmitter molecules are released. The molecules quickly diffuse across the synaptic cleft.

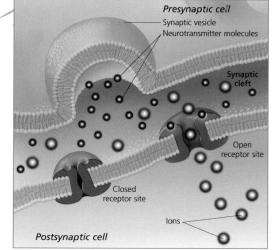

Presynaptic cell
Synaptic vesicle
Neurotransmitter molecules

Synaptic cleft

Open receptor site

Closed receptor site

Postsynaptic cell

Ions

Receptor sites

The post-synaptic cell membrane contains receptor proteins that act as gates or channels. Neurotransmitter molecules can bind with a receptor, opening a channel for specific ions. When enough ions have passed through the channel, the potential of the postsynaptic cell changes.

Axon terminal

Presynaptic cell

Neurotransmitter reuptake
Broken-down neurotransmitter

Enzyme

Neurotransmitter reuptake

Synaptic cleft

Ion

Postsynaptic cell

Axon terminal fiber

Transmitter secretion

Synaptic knob
(Or axon terminal of presynaptic neuron)

Removal of neurotransmitters

The effects of neurotransmitters are short-lived, because the cleft has to be cleared for future actions. The neurotransmitter molecules are either broken down by enzymatic action or reabsorbed and repackaged (*reuptake*).

PLATE 12

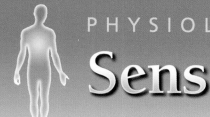

Sensory Receptors

What are sensory receptors?

Our ability to sense and respond to the environment includes **sensation**, the awareness of a stimulus, and **perception**, the understanding of the meaning of a stimulus. **Sensory receptors**, highly specialized nerve cells, help us detect light, temperature and other kinds of energy. These receptors **transduce**, or convert, the various types of energy into signals understood by the nervous system. Each type of receptor responds to a specific form of energy–rods & cones respond to light, and olfactory receptor cells to odorants (chemicals).

Connective tissue capsule
(lamellated disc in the skin)

Nerve ending · Axon · Nerve cell body · Terminal

Pressure sensor

Sensory nerves

An example of a sensory receptor is the Pacinian (lamellated) corpuscle, a mechanoreceptor in the skin that detects pressure and vibration. The lamellations cushion the dendrite against light touch, and spread the pressure around the dendrite. The capsule deforms (mechanical), increasing permeability and depolarizing the membrane, which generates a potential (electrical). If there is enough of a stimulus, a nerve impulse is generated.

Stimulus transduction

1 Applied pressure

Capsule deforms · Axon · Nerve cell

Nerve ending

2 Generation of impulse

3 Impulse transmission · Terminal

4 Impulse is sent to the brain

Receptor response

When a stimulus is strong enough to exceed the threshold potential, a nerve impulse is generated. If the stimulus gets stronger, the amplitude (size and strength) of the impulse stays the same, but the rate of impulse generation increases (more pressure, more impulses).

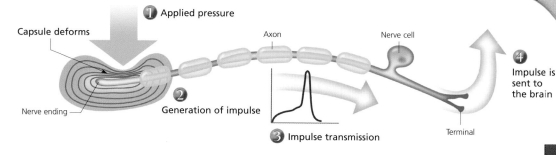

Pressure · Increasing pressure · Increasing pressure

Amplitude · Nerve impulses

Threshold potential

Time

Tactile discrimination

Through our sense of touch, we are able to distinguish, or discriminate, between various stimuli, such as different pressures or temperatures. We can judge the strength of a stimulus (intensity discrimination) and differentiate between locations of stimuli (spatial discrimination)

In the skin, the peripheral dendrites of a sensory neuron branch radially, producing a circular **receptive field**. Sensitivity is proportional to the number of receptive fields in a given area. When the fields are far apart, a stimulus affecting one area may not affect the field next to it. When the fields are close together, a stimulus would affect several fields at the same time.

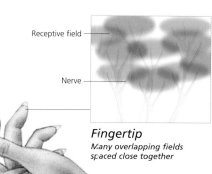

Receptive field · Nerve

Fingertip
Many overlapping fields spaced close together

Receptive field · Nerve

Back
Few fields spaced far apart

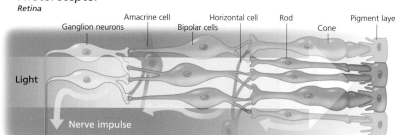

Skeletal muscle · Sensory nerve · Spindle (intrafusal) fibers

Mechanoreceptor
Muscle spindle

Receptor adaptation

Some receptors are **tonic**, or always active. Other receptors, known as **phasic**, only become active when there is a change in the stimulus. Receptor adaptation is a way of reducing sensitivity to a continued stimulus. Pressure and light touch receptors in the skin are fast adapting types. We are aware of our clothes when we put them on, but then we forget about the sensation. An example of slowly-adapting receptors are **proprioceptors**, mechanoreceptors that monitor joint position and muscle tension. Since pain generally signals a problem, **nociceptors** (pain receptors) show little adaptation.

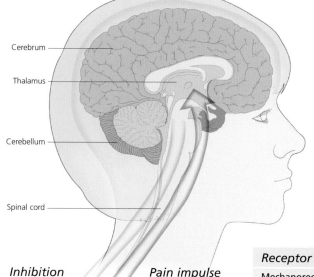

Cerebrum · Thalamus · Cerebellum · Spinal cord

Inhibition response · *Pain impulse*

Spinal cord

Sensory input

Sensory pathways

Pressure and proprioception sensations are carried by very long myelinated fibers up to the medulla oblongata (in the brainstem). The information is then passed through neurons to the thalamus. Temperature and pain sensations are carried by thin unmyelinated fibers to the spinal cord. Information is then passed through neurons in the spinal cord up to the thalamus. Centers in the brain stem can inhibit pain sensations by signalling through descending fibers, suppressing the relay of pain signals.

Photoreceptor
Retina

Ganglion neurons · Amacrine cell · Bipolar cells · Horizontal cell · Rod · Cone · Pigment layer

Light

Nerve impulse

Receptor types	Stimulus	Example
Mechanoreceptor	displacement & deformation	Light & heavy touch, pressure (the skin)
		Movement & balance (the inner ear)
		Joint position (throughout the body)
		Blood pressure (baroreceptor in aortic wall)
Thermoreceptor	temperature	Free nerve endings (the skin)
Chemoreceptor	chemical	Olfactory receptor cells (the sense of smell)
		Gustatory receptor cells (the sense of taste)
		Carotid & aortic bodies (detect oxygen in the blood)
Photoreceptor	light	Rods and cones (the retina of the eye)
Nociceptor	noxious stimuli/pain	Free nerve endings (the skin)

Chemoreceptor
Taste bud

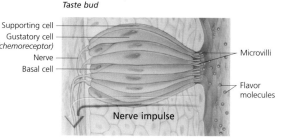

Supporting cell · Gustatory cell (chemoreceptor) · Nerve · Basal cell · Microvilli · Flavor molecules

Nerve impulse

PLATE 13

Hormonal Action

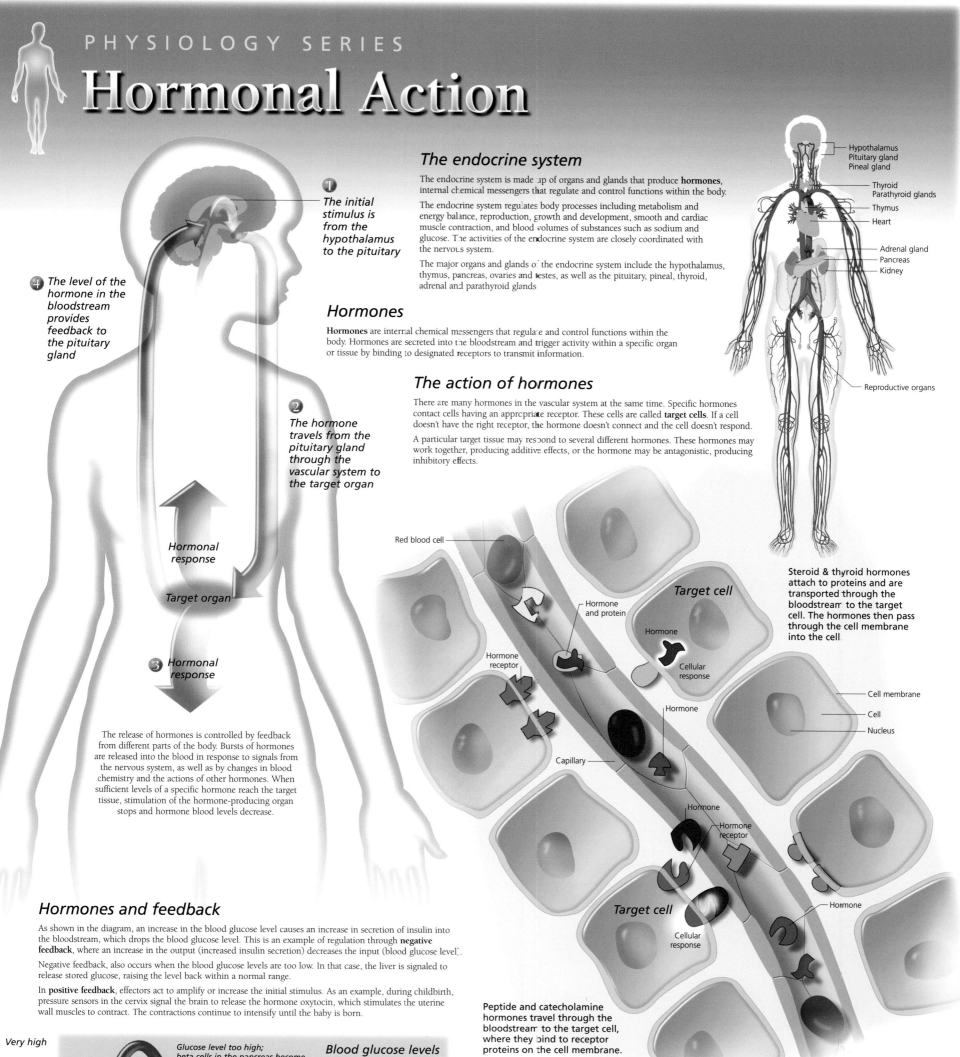

① The initial stimulus is from the hypothalamus to the pituitary

④ The level of the hormone in the bloodstream provides feedback to the pituitary gland

② The hormone travels from the pituitary gland through the vascular system to the target organ

Hormonal response

Target organ

③ Hormonal response

The release of hormones is controlled by feedback from different parts of the body. Bursts of hormones are released into the blood in response to signals from the nervous system, as well as by changes in blood chemistry and the actions of other hormones. When sufficient levels of a specific hormone reach the target tissue, stimulation of the hormone-producing organ stops and hormone blood levels decrease.

The endocrine system

The endocrine system is made up of organs and glands that produce **hormones**, internal chemical messengers that regulate and control functions within the body.

The endocrine system regulates body processes including metabolism and energy balance, reproduction, growth and development, smooth and cardiac muscle contraction, and blood volumes of substances such as sodium and glucose. The activities of the endocrine system are closely coordinated with the nervous system.

The major organs and glands of the endocrine system include the hypothalamus, thymus, pancreas, ovaries and testes, as well as the pituitary, pineal, thyroid, adrenal and parathyroid glands

Hormones

Hormones are internal chemical messengers that regulate and control functions within the body. Hormones are secreted into the bloodstream and trigger activity within a specific organ or tissue by binding to designated receptors to transmit information.

The action of hormones

There are many hormones in the vascular system at the same time. Specific hormones contact cells having an appropriate receptor. These cells are called **target cells**. If a cell doesn't have the right receptor, the hormone doesn't connect and the cell doesn't respond.

A particular target tissue may respond to several different hormones. These hormones may work together, producing additive effects, or the hormone may be antagonistic, producing inhibitory effects.

Hypothalamus
Pituitary gland
Pineal gland

Thyroid
Parathyroid glands
Thymus
Heart

Adrenal gland
Pancreas
Kidney

Reproductive organs

Red blood cell

Hormone and protein

Target cell

Hormone

Hormone receptor

Cellular response

Hormone

Capillary

Hormone

Steroid & thyroid hormones attach to proteins and are transported through the bloodstream to the target cell. The hormones then pass through the cell membrane into the cell

Cell membrane
Cell
Nucleus

Hormone

Hormone receptor

Target cell

Cellular response

Hormone

Peptide and catecholamine hormones travel through the bloodstream to the target cell, where they bind to receptor proteins on the cell membrane.

Hormones and feedback

As shown in the diagram, an increase in the blood glucose level causes an increase in secretion of insulin into the bloodstream, which drops the blood glucose level. This is an example of regulation through **negative feedback**, where an increase in the output (increased insulin secretion) decreases the input (blood glucose level).

Negative feedback, also occurs when the blood glucose levels are too low. In that case, the liver is signaled to release stored glucose, raising the level back within a normal range.

In **positive feedback**, effectors act to amplify or increase the initial stimulus. As an example, during childbirth, pressure sensors in the cervix signal the brain to release the hormone oxytocin, which stimulates the uterine wall muscles to contract. The contractions continue to intensify until the baby is born.

Very high

Glucose level

Normal range

Very low

Glucose level increases after a meal

Glucose level too high; beta cells in the pancreas become stimulated, releasing insulin

Blood glucose levels

Glucose level in normal range; homeostasis is restored

Glucose level decreases after insulin release

Glucose level too low; alpha cells in the pancreas become stimulated, signaling liver to release the stored glucose

Time

Examples of body functions & associated hormones

Gland	Hormone	Body function
Ovaries	Estrogen	Follicle (egg) maturation and sexual development
Pancreas	Insulin	Glucose uptake
Pineal	Melatonin	Body rhythms (sleep)
Pituitary:		
anterior	Growth hormone	Growth and tissue repair
posterior	Antidiuretic hormone	Water retention and vasoconstriction
Testes	Testosterone	Sexual development
Thyroid	Thyroxine	Overall metabolic rate

PLATE 15

CSF & The Brain

Support and protection of the brain

Cerebrospinal fluid (CSF) is a clear, watery liquid that circulates around and within the central nervous system (CNS). The brain is suspended inside the cranium in the fluid environment of CSF. Normally the brain weighs about 1,500 grams, but the CSF provides buoyancy, allowing the apparent weight of the brain to be about 50 grams. CSF acts as a shock absorber, spreading the force of an impact over a larger area. CSF also supplies nutrients to the neurons and glial cells, transports active biochemicals such as neurotransmitters and hormones, and removes waste products from the central nervous system.

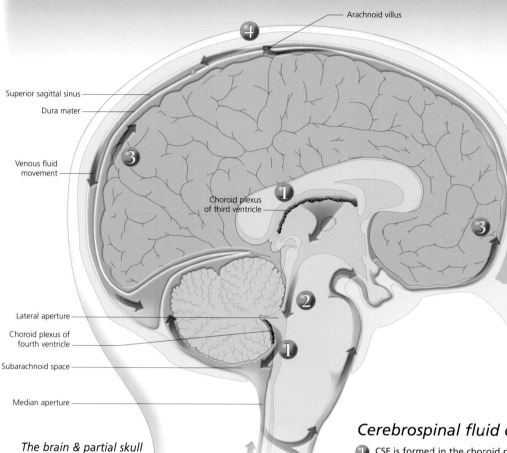

Arachnoid villus
Superior sagittal sinus
Dura mater
Venous fluid movement
Choroid plexus of third ventricle
Lateral aperture
Choroid plexus of fourth ventricle
Subarachnoid space
Median aperture

The brain & partial skull
(Sagittal section)

Cranial meninges

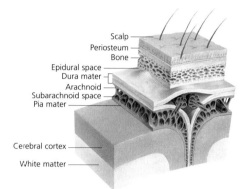

Scalp
Periosteum
Bone
Epidural space
Dura mater
Arachnoid
Subarachnoid space
Pia mater
Cerebral cortex
White matter

The brain is also protected by the **cranial meninges**, three layers of tissue that keep the brain from contacting the cranial bones. The meninges provide circulation of cerebrospinal fluid and carry blood vessels supplying blood to the brain. The outer layer, the **dura mater**, is fused to the cranial bone lining. The innermost layer, the **pia mater**, is attached to the surface of the brain. The middle layer, the **arachnoid mater**, contains a meshwork of elastic and collagen fibers (**arachnoid trabecula**). Within and supported by the meshwork are cerebral arteries and veins surrounded by CSF.

Arachnoid villus

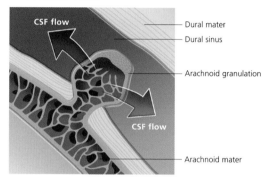

CSF flow
Dural mater
Dural sinus
Arachnoid granulation
CSF flow
Arachnoid mater

CSF reenters the venous system through the walls of **arachnoid granulations**, collections of villi or projections. The granulations protrude from the subarachnoid space into the superior sagittal sinus, allowing one-way transfer of cerebrospinal fluid into circulation.

Cerebrospinal fluid circulation

1. CSF is formed in the choroid plexus.
2. CSF flows from the choroid plexus into the ventricles and the central canal of the spinal cord.
3. CSF flows into subarachnoid space around the brain.
4. CSF reenters the venous system through the arachnoid granulations.

Choroid plexus and brain capillary

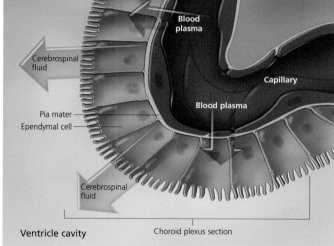

Blood plasma
Cerebrospinal fluid
Capillary
Blood plasma
Pia mater
Ependymal cell
Cerebrospinal fluid
Ventricle cavity
Choroid plexus section

CSF formation

Cerebrospinal fluid is mainly secreted by the choroid plexuses, specialized capillaries within the ventricles of the brain. CSF is a combination of an ultrafiltrate of blood and secretions of the ependymal cells lining the ventricles and central canal of the spinal cord. Cerebrospinal fluid is similar to blood plasma but contains more of hydrogen, magnesium, sodium and chloride ions and less potassium and calcium ions and glucose.

Ventricles of the brain
(Lateral view)

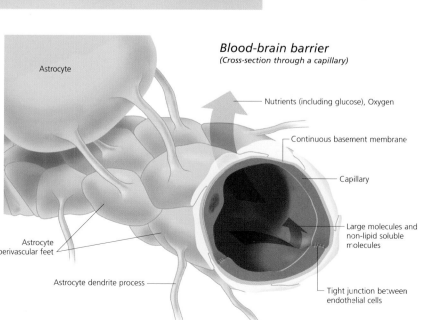

Lateral ventricle
A - Anterior horn
B - Posterior horn
C - Inferior horn
Interventricular foramina
Third ventricle
Cerebral aqueduct
Fourth ventricle
Lateral foramina
Medial foramen

The ventricles

The ventricles are CSF-filled cavities within the brain and brain stem. Each cerebral hemisphere has a lateral ventricle (first and second ventricles), connected through intraventricular foramina to the third ventricle, a smaller cavity in the middle of the brain. The cerebral or mesencephalic aqueduct connects the third and fourth ventricles. The fourth ventricle merges with the central canal of the spinal cord.

Blood-brain barrier
(Cross-section through a capillary)

Astrocyte
Nutrients (including glucose), Oxygen
Continuous basement membrane
Capillary
Astrocyte perivascular feet
Large molecules and non-lipid soluble molecules
Astrocyte dendrite process
Tight junction between endothelial cells

The blood-brain barrier

Hormones and other chemicals in the blood could disturb neural function, so the blood-brain barrier isolates neural tissue from the general circulation. The endothelial cells of the brain's capillaries are joined by tight junctions. The surfaces of the capillaries are mostly covered by extensions, or processes of **astrocytes**, a type of supporting cell in neural tissue. The combination of tight junctions and the astrocyte covering provides reduced permeability while still allowing passage of certain substances, like oxygen and glucose.

PLATE 16

Fluid Balance & Filtration

The urinary system

The urinary system is responsible for three major functions in the body: removing wastes, maintaining normal water volume, and controlling acid-base balance in the bloodstream. The individual components of the urinary system (bladder, kidneys, ureters and urethra) each play an important role in these processes.

Urine formation begins within tiny functional units of the kidneys called **nephrons**. A complex, three-step process of filtration, reabsorption and secretion removes metabolic wastes, allows important substances such as glucose and water to be passed back into the blood, and eliminates toxins such as drugs and ammonia. The filtrate that results from this process is eventually diluted with water to produce urine.

The urinary system

- Kidney
- Ureter
- Bladder
- Urethra

The kidney

The kidneys are located on each side of the spine at the back of the abdominal cavity. Each kidney is approximately 4 to 5 inches long and connects to the bladder via a narrow muscular tube called a **ureter**. We are normally born with a pair of kidneys; however, we can survive with a single kidney.

Within the kidney are two main regions. The outer rim is the **renal cortex**, which contains the **nephrons**, tiny microscopic units that filter blood (see below). The inner region is the **renal medulla**. It consists of many cone-shaped structures (**renal pyramids**) that transport urine to the **calyces**, cup-shaped cavities in the center of the kidney. The calyces drain into the **renal sinus**, a central chamber that connects directly to the ureter.

Kidney
(Sectioned view)

Labels: Renal fascia, Perirenal fat, Fibrous capsule, Renal papilla, Renal sinus, Major calyx, Minor calyx, Arcuate artery, Arcuate vein, Renal pyramid, Renal cortex, Renal medulla, Interlobar vein, Interlobar artery, Renal artery, Renal vein, Ureter, Urine

Blood flow

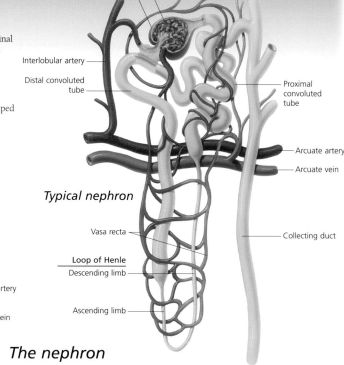

Typical nephron

Labels: Glomerulus, Glomerular capsule, Interlobular artery, Distal convoluted tube, Proximal convoluted tube, Arcuate artery, Arcuate vein, Collecting duct, Vasa recta

Loop of Henle
- Descending limb
- Ascending limb

The nephron

Each kidney contains more than a million **nephrons**, the microscopic units located in the outer renal cortex. A single nephron is made up of four components: the renal corpuscle, the proximal convoluted tubule, the loop of Henle and the distal convoluted tubule.

Glomerular capillary

Labels: Filtrate, Filtration slit, Podocyte, Blood pressure, Fenestration, Red blood cell, Pedicel, Protein, Filtrate, Blood flow

Filtration

As blood flows through the glomerular capillary, blood pressure exerts a force that pushes fluid and dissolved substances through the filtration apparatus. There are three parts to the apparatus: the capillary walls, the basement membrane and the glomerular epithelium. The pores in the fenestrated capillary are large enough to allow plasma and solutes to diffuse, but too small for blood cells to pass. The basement membrane (**lamina densa**) is thicker and more dense than a typical basement membrane. This allows smaller proteins and nutrients to pass but not larger proteins.

The outer surface of the basement membrane is surrounded with **podocytes**, specialized cells with long processes, or **pedicels**, that wrap around the membrane. The pedicels are separated by very narrow gaps called **filtration slits**. The combination of high fluid pressure, selectively permeable membranes and large filtration surface areas allows a large volume of fluid to be filtered.

How urine is produced

The kidneys process an average of 200 quarts of blood daily, eventually excreting only about 2 quarts of extra water and waste products as urine. Urine production begins when blood enters the nephrons. After a complex process of reabsorption and secretion along the renal tubule, concentrated urine containing water and wastes such as sodium and urea (a by-product of toxic ammonia products formed in the liver) leaves the collecting ducts.

Filtrate formation in the nephron

Labels: Blood flow, Afferent arteriole, Efferent arteriole, Glomerulus, Filtration, Water, Sodium and chlorine ions, Glucose, Proximal convoluted tube, Tubular reabsorption, Filtrate flow, Distal convoluted tube, Tubular reabsorption and secretion, Water, Blood flow, Potassium, Filtrate flow, Reabsorption, Water, Urea, Collecting tube, Sodium & chlorine ions, Urine flow, Excretion, Blood flow, Water

The composition of urine

- 5% solutes*
- 95% water

*(Solutes include urea, sodium, sulfate and phosphate ions, and uric acid)

Key stages of urine formation

- **Filtration** — Filtering of water, waste products, sodium, glucose and other chemicals
- **Reabsorption** — Movement of usable substances back to the bloodstream
- **Secretion** — Transport of waste materials from capillaries around the renal tubule back into the distal tubule for removal with the urine

ADH and fluid levels

Labels: Pituitary gland, Low fluid intake or excessive sweating, Blood volume drops, Pituitary gland secretes ADH, ADH secretion is inhibited, Collecting duct, ADH increases permeability of collecting ducts, Increased water absorption from increase in permeability, Blood volume increases, Urine volume decreases

ADH & fluid volume

ADH, or antidiuretic hormone, increases the permeability of the collecting ducts, which increases the reabsorbtion of water. ADH is produced in the hypothalamus and stored in the pituitary gland. The hypothalamus responds to changes in blood volume by changing the amount of ADH that is sent into the system. This is an example of a negative feedback process that helps to maintain blood volume levels within a certain range.

PLATE 17

Homeostasis & Heat Regulation

Homeostasis

Our external environment is constantly changing, presenting us with many physical stresses. In order to continue functioning, we need to maintain **homeostasis**, meaning a stable, constant internal environment.

When an internal condition, such as the blood glucose level or the body's core temperature, becomes too far from normal, mechanisms are activated to cause the condition to change so as to maintain homeostasis. After the condition is back within an acceptable range, the mechanisms are signaled to stop. Sending information back to modify a process is called **feedback**.

Feedback and homeostasis

An example of homeostasis and feedback occurs with blood glucose. An increase in the blood glucose level causes an increase in secretion of the hormone **insulin** into the bloodstream, which drops the blood glucose level. This is an example of regulation through **negative feedback**, where an increase in the output (increased insulin secretion) decreases the input (blood glucose level).

In **positive feedback**, effectors act to amplify or increase the initial stimulus. As an example, during childbirth, pressure sensors in the cervix signal the brain to release the hormone **oxytocin**, which stimulates the uterine wall muscles to contract. The contractions continue to intensify until the baby is born.

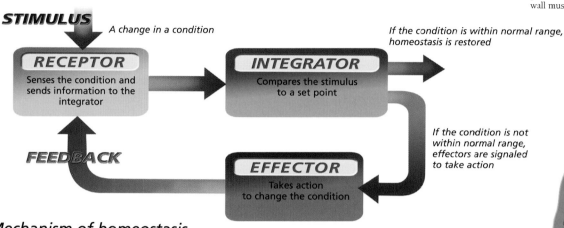

STIMULUS — A change in a condition

RECEPTOR — Senses the condition and sends information to the integrator

INTEGRATOR — Compares the stimulus to a set point

If the condition is within normal range, homeostasis is restored

If the condition is not within normal range, effectors are signaled to take action

FEEDBACK

EFFECTOR — Takes action to change the condition

Mechanism of homeostasis

Three interacting components provide a way to maintain the stability of our internal environment. **Receptors** sense internal and external conditions, sending the information to an **integrator**, which compares the information to a set point. If the condition is within an acceptable level, no action is taken and homeostasis is maintained.

If the condition is outside of an acceptable level, then **effectors** are signaled to provide a suitable response. The response changes the initial condition, and the receptor senses the change. The integrator again compares the information from the receptor to a set point, and, if necessary, signals effectors. This process continues until homeostasis is restored.

Body temperature

We generate heat internally (**endothermically**) through our **metabolism**, the sum total of all the chemical reactions in the body. Metabolism includes the processes of digestion, respiration and blood circulation. Each of the chemical reactions generates heat.

Homeostatic mechanisms keep our internal temperature relatively constant through changes in external temperatures.

Internal body heat

Heat transfer modes

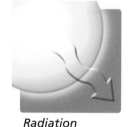

Radiation
Heat gain through exposure to radiant energy, such as sunlight

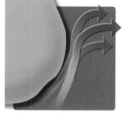

Convection
Air or water movement aids loss of heat into an environment

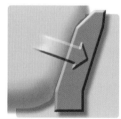

Conduction
Transfer of heat between the body and an object

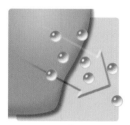

Evaporation
Conversion of a liquid (like sweat) into a gas (water vapor)

Skin

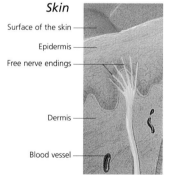

- Surface of the skin
- Epidermis
- Free nerve endings
- Dermis
- Blood vessel

Regulation of body temperature

Our behavior and body function change to adjust to heat gains and losses. Physiological mechanisms include changes in peripheral blood vessels and metabolism, while behavioral changes can involve clothing adjustments or moving to a different environment.

Receptors, such as free nerve endings in the skin, sense the external temperatures. The information is sent to the hypothalamus, the temperature regulation center in the brain. Effectors, like the smooth muscles around capillaries, are signaled by the hypothalamus to respond. When the hypothalamus is signaled (through feedback) that a suitable temperature has been reached, responses are stopped.

Brain
(Sagittal view)

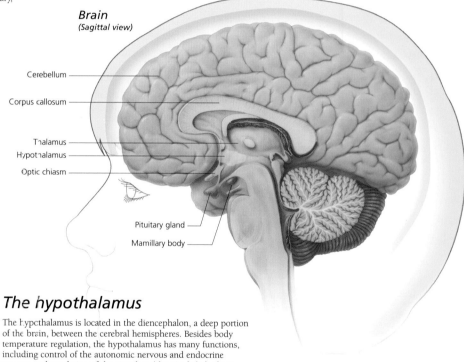

- Cerebellum
- Corpus callosum
- Thalamus
- Hypothalamus
- Optic chiasm
- Pituitary gland
- Mamillary body

The hypothalamus

The hypothalamus is located in the diencephalon, a deep portion of the brain, between the cerebral hemispheres. Besides body temperature regulation, the hypothalamus has many functions, including control of the autonomic nervous and endocrine systems and regulation of the circadian (sleep/wake) rhythms.

Response to heat

In a hot environment, we increase heat loss in several ways. The smooth muscles at the capillary junctions relax, and blood flows into the peripheral capillaries. Heat is transferred from the blood vessels, through the skin and into the outside environment. We also lose heat through increased sweating. Our metabolism may decrease, which reduces the internal generation of heat.

Behaviorally we can wear less clothing or looser clothing and move out of the sun. Putting on a fan or getting into water increases heat loss through convection.

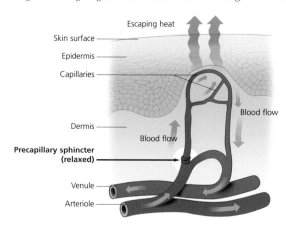

- Escaping heat
- Skin surface
- Epidermis
- Capillaries
- Blood flow
- Dermis
- Blood flow
- **Precapillary sphincter (relaxed)**
- Venule
- Arteriole

In a warmer environment

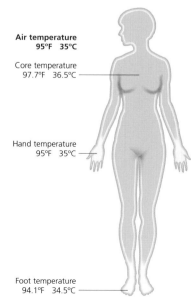

Air temperature
95°F 35°C

Core temperature
97.7°F 36.5°C

Hand temperature
95°F 35°C

Foot temperature
94.1°F 34.5°C

Response to cold

In a cold environment, we decrease heat loss in several ways. The smooth muscles at the capillary junctions contract, stopping the blood flow into the peripheral capillaries. Heat stays in the blood vessels, moving back into the body through the venous system. This helps to maintain a consistent core temperature. Our metabolism may increase, producing higher internal generation of heat.

Behaviorally we can put on more clothing, and sometimes make use of the heat of the sun. Staying out of the wind and water decreases heat loss through convection.

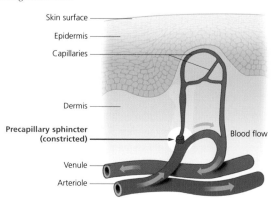

- Skin surface
- Epidermis
- Capillaries
- Dermis
- **Precapillary sphincter (constricted)**
- Blood flow
- Venule
- Arteriole

In a cooler environment

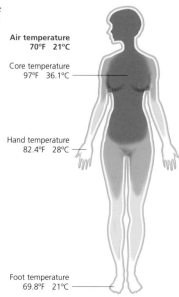

Air temperature
70°F 21°C

Core temperature
97°F 36.1°C

Hand temperature
82.4°F 28°C

Foot temperature
69.8°F 21°C

PLATE 19

Nutrition & Metabolism

What is nutrition?

Good nutrition is the cornerstone of human development and survival. **Nutrition** describes the process of how we consume, absorb and utilize **nutrients**, the substances in food that build tissue and provide energy. The six major types of nutrients are water, carbohydrates, proteins, fats, vitamins and minerals. Specific nutrients such as vitamin C, protein and certain amino acids are called **essential** because they are fundamental to health but cannot be manufactured by the body. Essential nutrients must be consumed in the diet.

Basal metabolic rate

The **basal metabolic rate** (BMR) is the amount of energy used while a person is in a resting state. BMR is determined by age, gender and size, and is strongly influenced by the thyroid gland.

The sum of the basal metabolic rate and the energy used by a person during their daily activities is the **total metabolic rate**. If the energy value (in calories) of ingested nutrients equals the total metabolic rate, then body weight doesn't change. When food intake is less than the total metabolic rate, then body weight goes down. Conversely body weight goes up when food intake exceeds the total metabolic rate.

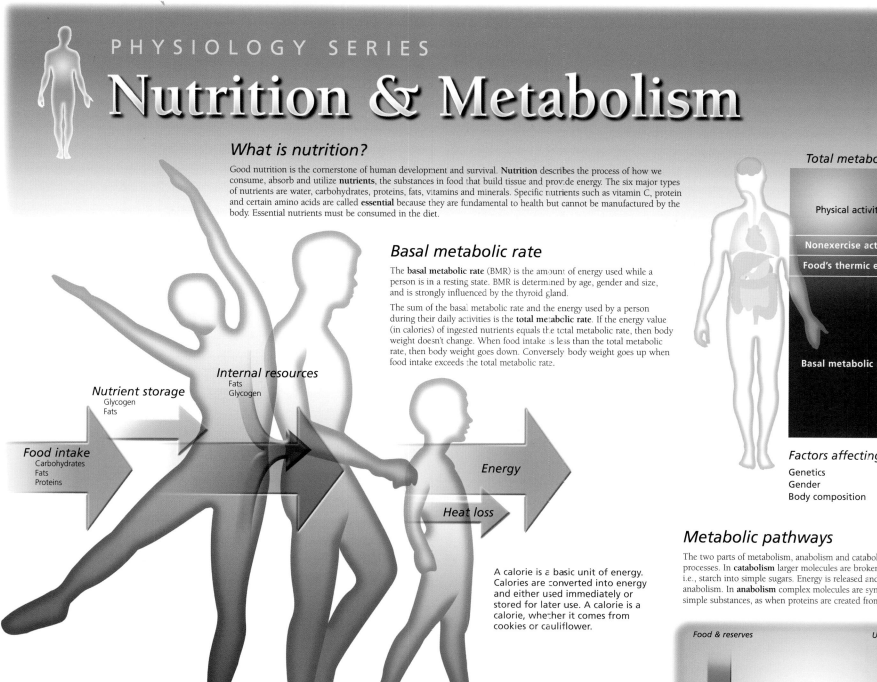

Nutrient storage
Glycogen
Fats

Internal resources
Fats
Glycogen

Food intake
Carbohydrates
Fats
Proteins

Energy

Heat loss

A calorie is a basic unit of energy. Calories are converted into energy and either used immediately or stored for later use. A calorie is a calorie, whether it comes from cookies or cauliflower.

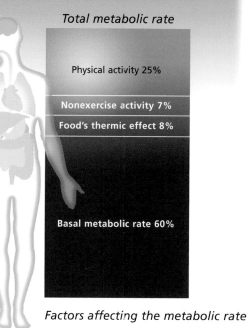

Total metabolic rate

Physical activity 25%

Nonexercise activity 7%

Food's thermic effect 8%

Basal metabolic rate 60%

Factors affecting the metabolic rate

Genetics	Level of activity
Gender	Age
Body composition	Hormonal action

Metabolic pathways

The two parts of metabolism, anabolism and catabolism, are complementary processes. In **catabolism** larger molecules are broken down into smaller ones, i.e., starch into simple sugars. Energy is released and captured for use by anabolism. In **anabolism** complex molecules are synthesized from more simple substances, as when proteins are created from amino acids.

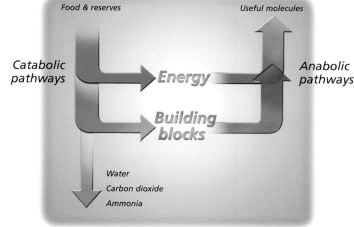

Food & reserves

Useful molecules

Catabolic pathways

Anabolic pathways

Energy

Building blocks

Water

Carbon dioxide

Ammonia

What is metabolism?

The foods and beverages we consume provide both energy (calories) and nutrients to support all of the body's organs and systems. They also protect against health risks and diseases and enable the body to maintain and repair itself. Nutrients are broken down into more simple substances by chemicals called **enzymes** in the digestive system. These substances are then transformed into the specific materials necessary for our survival.

Metabolism is the sum total of all the chemical reactions in the body. Besides the visible examples of muscle action and heat regulation, metabolism includes the processes of digestion, respiration, blood circulation and nervous system function. The **metabolic rate** describes the amount of energy we use over a certain period of time.

Food metabolism

Food is broken down by digestive enzymes into components small enough to be absorbed. Simple sugars (from carbohydrates) and amino acids (from proteins) enter the capillaries on their way to the portal vein, while absorbed fats enter the lymphatic vessels of the intestinal villi. These compounds make up the basic materials for metabolism. The common measurement of a food's energy value is a **kilocalorie** (C), equal to 1,000 calories.

Protein metabolism

Proteins are broken down into small **peptides** (chains of amino acids) and amino acids. 20 amino acids are necessary for good health, but we can only produce 11 on our own. The remaining 9 (the **essential amino acids**) must be supplied by the diet.

Proteins help build and repair tissue, speed up chemical reactions (as enzymes) and help make compounds like myosin (in muscle fibers) and hemoglobin (in red blood cells).

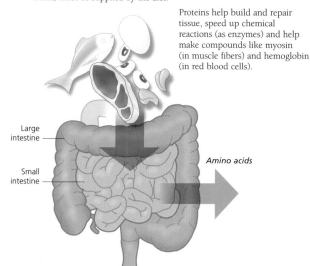

Large intestine

Small intestine

Amino acids

Carbohydrate metabolism

Intestinal enzymes break carbohydrates down into **monosaccharides** (simple sugars). The sugars, principally glucose, galactose and fructose, travel via the portal vein to the liver.

Hepatocytes (liver cells) convert the galactose and fructose into glucose, the only sugar normally found in blood. Unused glucose is stored in the liver as glycogen.

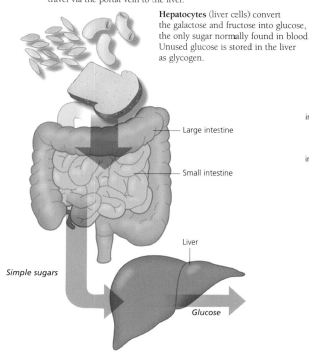

Large intestine

Small intestine

Simple sugars

Liver

Glucose

Fat metabolism

Fats are broken down into glycerol and fatty acids. Three particular fatty acids (essential fatty acids) must be supplied through the diet.

Fats used for fuel are stored in adipose tissue. Structural fats (cholesterol and phospholipids) are used for cell membranes and for synthesis of steroid hormones and vitamin D.

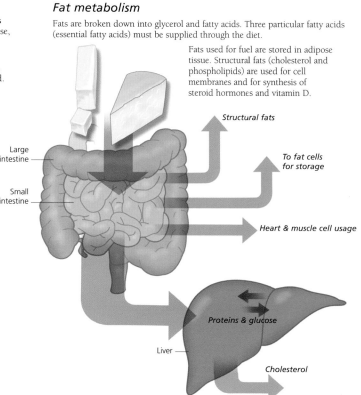

Structural fats

To fat cells for storage

Large intestine

Small intestine

Heart & muscle cell usage

Proteins & glucose

Liver

Cholesterol

PLATE 20